The Galveston Diet:

Transform Your Health with Delicious Recipes and Hormone-Balancing Strategies

By

Dr Albert M. Brose

Disclaimer page

As you read through these pages, remember that there is a surprise at the conclusion of this book—a Free Gift to help you on your health journey even further. Thank you for coming on this transforming journey with us!"

Table of contents

INTRODUCTION

Unveiling the Galveston Diet: Your Path to Thriving, Younger You

Have you ever felt as if your body was working against you? Fatigue, obstinate weight gain, and a constant fog clouding your thoughts are just a few murmurs from a symphony of hormonal imbalance taking place inside. For far too many of us, they become unpleasant companions, serving as frequent reminders that something is wrong. But what if there was a way to tone down the discordant notes and create a lovely song of vigorous health?

The Galveston Diet is more than simply a collection of recipes or stringent guidelines. It is a transforming movement, a concept that allows you to take control of your own well-being. It's about learning the language your hormones use and using that knowledge to create a symphony of sustenance and life.

Imagine waking up every day with a newfound enthusiasm for life. Or having a spring in your step and a keen, concentrated mind. Imagine putting on clothing that used to feel restrictive but is now a representation of your confident, healthy self. This is not a faraway fantasy; it is the reality that awaits you on the other side of the Galveston Diet.

This book is your unique road map to completing this transition. We'll dig into the intriguing science of hormones, discovering their enormous effects on our metabolism, emotions, and general health. You'll learn about the Galveston Diet's unique approach, which is a symphony of tasty, nutrient-dense meals meant to restore your hormonal orchestra to perfect harmony.

We'll look at inflammation, the silent cause of so many health issues, and give you the skills you need to quiet its disturbing murmurs. But this adventure goes far beyond your plate. We'll look at the benefits of mindful eating and how to have a long-term relationship with food that feeds both your body and your spirit.

The Galveston Diet is not a one-size-fits-all plan. Whether you want to lose weight, manage hormonal changes like perimenopause, or just improve your health, this book gives you the foundation and freedom to create a strategy that works for you. We'll look at ways to tailor your diet and overcome dietary constraints.

Your journey to robust health will not be linear; there will be moments of victory and missteps along the road. But don't worry, you're not alone on this trip. We'll look at the relationship between exercise, sleep, stress management, and general well-being, taking a comprehensive approach to creating a symphony of health that echoes throughout your life.

By the time you finish this book, you'll have the information, tasty recipes, and steadfast confidence to go on a transforming journey. You'll be ready to transform the whispers of discord into a resounding chorus of vigor, demonstrating your amazing potential. Are you prepared to begin? Let us flip the page and create the symphony of your vibrant health.

Chapter 1: Understanding Hormones and Their Impact on Our Wellbeing: The Body's Orchestra of Chemical Messengers

Imagine your body as a beautiful orchestra. Each organ, a skilled artist, plays a crucial part in the symphony of health. But to achieve balance, they need a director – a set of chemical signals called hormones. When these messages are in sync, the music is beautiful, a peak of energy and well-being. But when their voices become disjointed, the music falters, replaced by a depressing medley of symptoms.

For many of us, this imbalance appears as a nagging sense of disease. The unexpected weight gain, the tiredness that sticks to us despite ample sleep, the low mood that casts a long shadow – these are just a few signs that the hormonal orchestra is out of tune. But knowing these messages and their impact is the first step to reclaiming the conductor's baton and creating a song of vibrant health.

Our bodies make a variety of hormones, each having a specific role. Insulin controls blood sugar, keeping our energy levels steady. Estrogen and progesterone organize the monthly period and affect mood. Testosterone fuels sex drive and muscle growth. The thyroid hormone, the master of metabolism, determines how quickly we burn calories. These are just a few examples, and the relationship between them is nothing short of interesting.

Think of hormones like whispers, carrying information throughout the body. They move through the bloodstream, docking onto receptors on our cells, causing a chain of events. When these messages are given exactly and read correctly, our bodies work beautifully. But when hormone production is interrupted, or cellular receptors become immune, the messages get jumbled, leading to a symphony of disharmony.

This chemical imbalance can be caused by different causes. Chronic stress, a merciless director barking out frantic orders, can break the delicate balance. Age, like a slow lowering of the lights, can lead to a decrease in hormone release. Diet, the quality of the fuel we provide our instruments, can also play a major role. An excess of processed foods and sugary treats can cause inflammation, a constant heckler in the crowd, putting the entire show into confusion.

The good news is that we can affect the endocrine music. In the next chapter, we'll dive into the Galveston Diet, a unique method meant to bring your hormonal orchestra back into perfect balance. We'll explore how delicious, nutrient-rich foods can act as strong modulators, coaxing your hormones to sing their sweetest song. By knowing the language of hormones and handling the stick of thoughtful eating, you can become the director of your own well-being, creating a song of health that echoes for years to come.

Chapter 2: The Galveston Diet: A Comprehensive Approach to Hormonal Harmony - A Culinary Crescendo for Your Wellbeing

Imagine entering a symphony hall where the orchestra is in perfect harmony. The violins soar, the cellos vibrate, and the instruments merge together in a lovely tapestry of sound. This, my friends, is the core of the Galveston Diet — a symphony of delectable, nutrient-rich meals meant to put your hormonal orchestra into perfect harmony.

Unlike typical diets that concentrate exclusively on calorie restriction, the Galveston Diet takes a comprehensive approach. We believe that genuine change emerges from feeding your body at a cellular level, supplying the essential building blocks it needs to perform efficiently. By combining these concepts, you'll be wielding the conductor's baton, orchestrating a symphony of health that vibrates throughout your whole self.

The cornerstone of the Galveston Diet depends on two pillars: anti-inflammatory foods and intermittent fasting. Chronic, low-grade inflammation — a hidden saboteur hiding inside many of us – impairs hormone communication. The Galveston Diet confronts this head-on by integrating a vivid palette of anti-inflammatory superstars. Think of them as the tranquil melody that relaxes the symphony, enabling each instrument to play at its best.

These anti-inflammatory powerhouses include: Colorful fruits and vegetables: Packed with antioxidants, they quench the free radical fires that can damage cells and contribute to inflammation. Healthy fats: Avocados, nuts, and fatty fish are rich in omega-3 fatty acids, renowned for their anti-inflammatory properties. Lean protein sources: Grass-fed beef, poultry, and lentils give the building blocks for cellular repair and hormone synthesis.

Intermittent fasting, the second pillar of the Galveston Diet, functions as a conductor's repose, enabling your body to concentrate on regeneration. By intelligently compressing your eating window, you convert your body's metabolism into fat-burning mode, improving hormonal balance and general well-being.

But the Galveston Diet isn't just about restriction; it's about celebration. We've produced a treasure trove of tasty recipes, converting ordinary meals into gourmet masterpieces that delight your taste buds while nourishing your body. Imagine delicious fish drenched in a vivid herb sauce, a symphony of flavors that satisfies your palette while encouraging healthy inflammation levels. Or envision a dish brimming with antioxidant-rich berries topped with creamy yogurt — a delectable treat that helps hormonal balance.

The brilliance of the Galveston Diet resides in its versatility. We know that one size does not fit all. In the following chapter, we'll go into modifying the strategy to your individual requirements and tastes. Whether you're a busy professional seeking efficient meal prep tactics or someone with special dietary limitations, we'll empower you with the skills to build a personal symphony of health that resonates with your lifestyle. But before we dig further, know this: The Galveston Diet is more than simply a collection of recipes; it's a philosophy, a means of sustaining oneself from the inside out. It's about being the conductor of your own well-being, and the music you make will be a magnificent monument to the bright health that is inside you.

Chapter 3: Inflammation: The Unseen Disrupter Orchestrating Your Health Symphony

Imagine a symphony hall where a persistent cough disturbs the performance. It throws off the time, disturbs the musicians, and reduces the whole experience. This, my friends, is a metaphor for inflammation, a quiet culprit hiding inside many of us, upsetting the wonderful symphony of our health.

Inflammation, in its acute phase, is a normal reaction to injury or illness. It's the symphony in overdrive, pushing all its instruments into a frenzy to repair and defend. But when this acute inflammation becomes chronic, it's like that persistent cough that remains long after the illness is gone. It causes a low-grade buzz of disturbance throughout the body, wreaking havoc on our hormonal symphony and our entire well-being.

The reality is, that inflammation may lie in plain sight. You may not always feel the classic indicators of redness, swelling, or discomfort.

But behind the surface, it may be the silent conductor, throwing off the delicate balance of hormones and leading to a cascade of health concerns.

Let's look into the sneaky ways inflammation affects our hormonal homeostasis. One of its key targets is insulin, the maestro of blood sugar management. Chronic inflammation may lead to insulin resistance, a disease where your cells become deaf to insulin's instructions. This may spark a domino effect, leading to blood sugar abnormalities and a hormonal cascade that alters everything from metabolism to mood.

Inflammation also interrupts the sex hormone symphony. In women, it may worsen estrogen dominance, a condition associated with irregular periods, weight gain, and mood changes. In males, it may contribute to reduced testosterone levels, leading to weariness, decreased muscular mass, and a drop in libido.

But worry not, because the good news is that we can quiet the inflammatory chorus and restore harmony to our hormonal symphony. The Galveston Diet, presented in the last chapter, is a significant instrument in this struggle. By concentrating on anti-inflammatory foods, we can turn down the volume on this hidden disrupter.

These anti-inflammatory all-stars are more than simply dietary components; they're the instruments of a revolutionary symphony:

Leafy green vegetables: Powerhouses of antioxidants and phytonutrients, they temper the inflammatory fire.

Fatty fish: Rich in omega-3 fatty acids, these natural anti-inflammatory superstars help decrease inflammation throughout the body. Colorful fruits: Packed with antioxidants, they quench the free radical fires that lead to inflammation.

Herbs & spices: Don't overlook these tasty additions. Turmeric, ginger, and garlic contain significant anti-inflammatory effects.

However, the Galveston Diet goes beyond merely eating these anti-inflammatory nutrients. In the following chapter, we'll examine the power of mindful eating and developing a sustainable relationship with food. By knowing how your body reacts to various foods and creating a sense of intuitive eating, you may further silence the inflammatory voices and become the conductor of your own robust health. Remember, the path to optimum health is a beautiful symphony, and by knowing the role inflammation plays, you can guarantee that every note resonates with harmony and well-being.

Chapter 4: Delicious Recipe Makeovers: Turning Everyday Meals into Culinary Symphony

Let's face it: healthy eating is generally associated with dull salads and cooked veggies. But what if I told you that fuelling your body with wonderful, anti-inflammatory foods may be a symphony of taste and satisfaction? The Galveston Diet is not about deprivation; rather, it is about a culinary metamorphosis, an opportunity to convert your regular meals into masterpieces that delight your taste senses while directing your hormones toward beautiful harmony.

In this chapter, we'll go on a culinary expedition, revisiting some traditional recipes and giving them a Galveston Diet makeover. We'll replace inflammatory substances with anti-inflammatory alternatives while maintaining taste. Prepare to learn that healthy eating can be both a colorful burst of flavor and a monument to your dedication to your health.

From Bland Breakfast to Balanced Brilliance: The Scrambled Egg Revolution.

Many individuals eat fatty sausage and processed morning pastries, thereby setting the incorrect tone for their hormonal orchestra. However, with a simple change, you can turn your breakfast into a symphony of protein, healthy fats, and phytonutrients. Here's a recipe to help you get started.

Ingredients for Anti-Inflammatory Scrambled Eggs with Spinach, Sun-Dried Tomatoes, and Goat Cheese: 2 large eggs 1 tablespoon coconut oil ½ cup chopped spinach ¼ cup chopped sun-dried tomatoes 2 tablespoons crumbled goat cheese Salt and pepper to taste.

Instructions: In a bowl, whisk together the eggs. Heat the coconut oil in a skillet over medium heat.

Sauté the spinach until wilted.

Cook for one more minute after adding the sun-dried tomatoes.

Add the egg mixture and scramble until done. Sprinkle the goat cheese over top and season with salt and pepper.

This dish is full of taste and anti-inflammatory benefits. The spinach has vitamins and antioxidants, while the sun-dried tomatoes offer an acidic flavor. The goat cheese adds a creamy contrast to the fluffy eggs, and the healthful fats from the coconut oil keep you full all morning.

From Bland Pasta to Vibrant Veggie Delight: Weeknight Dinner Makeover

Pasta evenings may be a war between convenience vs health. But the Galveston Diet eliminates the necessity for compromise. Here's a dish that's as simple to make as your favorite boxed pasta but packed with taste and anti-inflammatory benefits:

Ingredients for Zucchini Noodle Primavera with Burst Cherry Tomatoes and Pine Nuts: - 2 medium zucchini noodles - 1 tablespoon olive oil - 1 minced garlic clove - ½ cup cherry tomatoes - ½ cup chopped asparagus - ¼ cup chopped broccoli florets - ¼ cup sliced red onion - ¼ cup chopped fresh basil - 2 tablespoons toasted pine nuts - Salt and pepper to taste Instructions: Use a spiralizer or julienne peeler to make zucchini noodles. In a pan over medium heat, warm the olive oil. Sauté garlic for 30 seconds, then add cherry tomatoes and simmer until bursting. Cook the asparagus, broccoli, and red onion until tender-crisp.

Add zucchini noodles and simmer for another 2-3 minutes until cooked through. Season with salt and pepper after stirring in the basil and pine nuts.

This dish is a harmonious blend of textures and tastes. The zucchini noodles provide a comforting basis, while the cherry tomatoes give a flash of flavor. The asparagus and broccoli provide a satisfying crunch, while the red onion provides a hint of sharpness. The pine nuts provide a nutty richness, while the fresh basil fills the dish with its fragrant flavor.

This is just a sample of the delightful changes you can make with the Galveston Diet. In the next chapter, we'll go over meal planning tactics to keep your taste buds satisfied and your health objectives on track. Remember that developing a sustainable relationship with food is an important aspect of the process. By adopting these anti-inflammatory changes into your daily routine, you'll be well on your way to creating a symphony of bright health, one delicious meal at a time.

Chapter 5: Meal Planning for Success: Practical Strategies for Busy Lives—Conducting Your Culinary Symphony with Ease

Life in the contemporary world is a stunning symphony of responsibilities. Juggling work, family, and personal activities may make us feel like we're always behind the conductor's stand, trying to keep up with the speed. But when it comes to fueling your body with the Galveston Diet's anti-inflammatory pleasures, there's no need for last-minute improvisation. With a little forethought and some creative tactics, you can turn meal preparation into a seamless part of your routine, ensuring that every note in your nutritional symphony rings out with delightful ease.

Here is the truth. Planning your meals does not have to be a time-consuming task. By devoting an hour or two each week, you may plan out a week's worth of nutritious, fulfilling meals. Consider it as preparing the stage for your culinary performance, ensuring that you have all of the necessary instruments (ingredients) to produce a masterpiece.

Here are some practical methods to transform meal planning into a stress-free symphony.

Embrace Batch Cooking: Complete a large amount of your week's meals in one sitting. This may include preparing chopped veggies, heating a big pot of protein, such as quinoa or chicken breasts, or making a double batch of a favorite soup. Having these pre-cooked ingredients on hand makes putting up dinners for the week a snap.

Befriend the Freezer: Not everything has to be consumed fresh. Soups, stews, and casseroles are stored exceptionally well, enabling you to reap the advantages of bulk cooking even on the busiest days. Individual portions are ideal for fast weeknight meals or grab-and-go lunches.

Get the Family Involved: Meal planning does not have to be done alone. Involve your family in the process by assigning chores such as recipe selection and shopping list creation. This not only fosters a feeling of ownership and responsibility, but it may also stimulate discussions about good eating habits.

Let's put these methods to use with an example meal plan for a busy week:

Sunday: Meal Planning and Preparation Day.

Spend 1-2 hours planning your meals for the week. For ideas, go through the book's recipe section or search online. Consider your schedule and choose fast and simple dinners for hectic weeknights.

Make a shopping list based on your preferred recipes. Include any essentials you currently have on hand, but prioritize the fresh foods you'll need for the week.

Do some batch cooking! Roast a pan of veggies, cook a pot of quinoa, or make a huge stir-fry foundation that can be used for numerous meals throughout the week.

Monday: Breakfast: Overnight Oats with Berries and Chia Seeds (prepared on Sunday).

Lunch: leftover stir-fry with grilled chicken Dinner: salmon with roasted asparagus and lemon butter sauce (recipe provided)

Tuesday: Breakfast: Scrambled Eggs with Spinach and Smoked Salmon (Recipe in Chapter 4).

Lunch: Lentil Soup (made on Sunday) with a side salad Dinner: Chicken Fajitas with sautéed peppers and onions, whole-wheat tortillas, and guacamole

Wednesday: Breakfast: Greek yogurt with berries and sliced almonds Lunch: Quinoa dish with roasted veggies and chickpeas (leftovers from Sunday) Dinner: Vegetarian chili with brown rice

Thursday (Repeat Monday or Tuesday meals):
Busy weeks happen! Do not be disheartened if you don't have time to cook every night. Having a pre-cooked alternative from earlier in the week helps you to keep a healthy habit while saving time.

Friday: Breakfast: Smoothie with Greek yogurt, spinach, banana, and protein powder Lunch: Leftover Chicken Fajitas from Tuesday Dinner: Takeout! Choose a restaurant that serves healthful dishes such as grilled salmon or lean protein with roasted veggies.

Saturday: Breakfast: Whole-wheat pancakes with fresh fruit and maple syrup.   Lunch: Leftover vegetarian chili from Wednesday. Dinner: Be creative! This is an excellent night to try out a new dish from the book or discover a different ethnic food.

This is just an example meal plan. Feel free to make changes according to your tastes, dietary requirements, and available time. The goal is to choose a strategy that is suitable for you and your lifestyle.

As you begin on this path of mindful eating and delightful changes, remember that the Galveston Diet is not about strict restrictions or calorie control. It's about building a lasting connection with food.

Chapter 6: Cultivating Mindful Eating Habits for Lasting Change - Conducting Your Symphony of Nourishment with Awareness

We've investigated the delightful wonders of the Galveston Diet, converting regular meals into culinary masterpieces that tickle your taste buds and nurture your health. We've gone into the science of inflammation, the quiet saboteur hiding inside, and uncovered the potential of anti-inflammatory foods to restore harmony to your hormonal symphony. But genuine change spreads beyond the plate. It entails building a thoughtful connection with food, a deep understanding of how you fuel yourself, and the emotions that drive your decisions.

Mindful eating is the conductor's baton in the symphony of your health. It's about approaching food with purpose, relishing each mouthful, and knowing how your body reacts to what you eat. It's about overcoming the autopilot mentality of thoughtless eating and entering into the present moment, enjoying the process of nutrition as a kind of self-care.

Here are some strategies to establish mindful eating habits and produce a permanent transformation:

Embrace the stop: Before each meal, spend a few seconds to stop and connect with your body. Ask yourself whether you're actually hungry or if you're grabbing food due to boredom, stress, or emotional triggers.

Practice thankfulness: Cultivate an attitude of thankfulness for the food on your plate. Consider the trip it made – from farm to table – and enjoy the nutrients it gives.

Slow Down and Savor: Put down your phone, turn off the TV, and establish a distraction-free atmosphere for your meals. Focus on the act of eating, appreciating the textures, smells, and fragrances of each mouthful. Chew deeply, enabling your body to register satiety signals.

Identify Emotional Eating Triggers: We all have them - those events or feelings that unconsciously urge us to go for unhealthy options. Recognize your triggers and build coping techniques. Perhaps it's a stroll in nature, a call to a friend, or a few deep breaths to handle stress instead of a bag of chips.

Embrace Imperfections: This trip is a lovely work in progress, not a strict quest for perfection. There will be days when you stumble, days when desires take control. Forgive yourself, learn from the experience, and recommit to mindful eating the following day.

Mindful eating isn't just about the meal itself; it's about fostering a feeling of self-awareness and compassion. By quieting the surrounding noise and listening to your internal signals, you become the conductor of your eating experience. You may pick healthful meals that connect with your body's requirements, and relish the process of eating as a kind of self-love.

In the following chapter, we'll discuss how to modify the Galveston Diet to your individual requirements and tastes. Whether you want to control weight, negotiate hormonal fluctuations, or just maximize your health, we'll give you the skills to build a customized symphony of nutrients. But before we dig further, know this: Cultivating mindful eating habits is a transforming gift you offer to yourself. It's about nurturing a profound appreciation for the food that feeds you and the body that takes you through life's tremendous journey. With each attentive mouthful, you create a symphony of self-care that echoes well beyond the plate.

Chapter 7: Achieving Weight Management and Sustainable Energy Levels: A Symphony of Balance and Vitality

For many of us, weight control and maintained energy levels seem like unreachable goals. The scales may appear to tilt persistently in the wrong way, while exhaustion throws a lengthy shadow over our days. But what if I told you that these challenges are typically based on the discord of your hormonal orchestra? By learning how the Galveston Diet tackles these imbalances, you may unleash the potential for healthy weight control, robust vitality, and a restored enthusiasm for life.

Crash diets and severe calorie restriction may offer rapid cures, but they typically leave us feeling starved and exhausted. The Galveston Diet offers a different approach. We concentrate on fueling your body with anti-inflammatory foods that support hormonal balance, naturally leading to good weight control and maintained energy levels.

Let's look into the science underlying this profound connection:

Insulin Harmony: Chronic inflammation affects insulin sensitivity, the key that unlocks your cells' capacity to absorb sugar from the circulation. When insulin activity is disrupted, blood sugar levels increase, causing the storage of extra calories as fat. The Galveston Diet, with its concentration on anti-inflammatory whole foods, helps restore insulin sensitivity, supporting balanced blood sugar levels and a more efficient metabolism.

Hormonal Harmony for Weight Management: Hormones like leptin and ghrelin play a critical role in controlling appetite and fullness. When inflammation alters these hormones, it may lead to increased cravings and trouble feeling satiated, making weight control a continual uphill fight. The Galveston Diet, by supporting hormonal balance, may help manage your appetite naturally, helping you to feel fuller for longer and make intuitive decisions regarding food.

Energy from Balanced Hormones: When your hormones are out of sync, it may wreak havoc on your energy levels. Imbalanced cortisol, the stress hormone, may contribute to weariness and sluggishness. The Galveston Diet integrates stress-management practices and supports good sleep patterns, both of which contribute to cortisol control and sustained energy throughout the day.

But the Galveston Diet isn't a magic bullet. It demands dedication and an adjustment in mentality. Here are some practical techniques to attain weight control and lasting energy with the Galveston Diet:

Focus on Nutrient Density: Prioritize entire, unprocessed meals full of vitamins, minerals, and fiber. These meals keep you feeling satiated, control blood sugar levels, and supply the building blocks for proper hormone activity.

Intermittent Fasting: Strategically compressing your eating window may be a great tool for weight control and cellular restoration. By adding intermittent fasting concepts into your practice, you may raise insulin sensitivity, stimulate fat burning, and enhance cellular health, leading to sustained energy levels.

Prioritize Sleep: Aim for 7-8 hours of decent sleep each night. Sleep deprivation alters hormones that govern appetite and fullness, making it difficult to manage weight and sustain energy levels.

Move Your Body: Regular physical exercise is a cornerstone of weight control and general well-being. Exercise helps manage blood sugar levels, increases insulin sensitivity, and enhances energy levels. Find activities you love, whether it's dancing, swimming, or brisk walking.

The path to attaining weight control and sustained energy levels is a lovely symphony, and the Galveston Diet gives the sheet music for a harmonic performance. It's about supporting your body with the correct meals, listening to its signs, and building healthy habits that become second nature.

In the following chapter, we'll investigate how to modify the Galveston Diet for your individual requirements. Whether you're undergoing hormonal fluctuations like perimenopause or have special dietary limitations, we'll provide you with the skills to develop a symphonic approach to health that resonates with your own requirements. Remember, successful weight control and robust vitality aren't about deprivation; it's about empowerment. It's about being the conductor of your own well-being, and the Galveston Diet is here to help you every step of the way.

Chapter 8: Navigating Perimenopause and Menopause with the Galveston Diet: A Symphony of Harmony Through Life's Transitions

For many women, perimenopause and menopause can feel like a jarring sound in the beautiful music of life. The once-harmonious hormonal orchestra explodes into a chaos of hot flashes, night sweats, sleep problems, and mood swings. But what if I told you that the Galveston Diet can be your conductor's baton, helping you arrange a symphony of well-being throughout these biological transitions?

Perimenopause, the years leading up to menopause, is a time of slow biological decline. Estrogen and progesterone, the lead musicians in your hormonal orchestra, begin to take a backseat, leading to a flurry of changes. These chemical changes can wreak havoc on your metabolism, sleep habits, and mental well-being.

Menopause itself, the final end of menstruation, is often presented as a bad event. But with the right attitude, it can be a time of strength and self-discovery. The Galveston Diet enables you to take care of your health during this shift, giving you the tools to handle these changes with grace and energy.

Let's dive into the specific ways the Galveston Diet can help you manage perimenopause and menopause:

Taming the Flames of Hot Flashes: Hot flashes, a hallmark sign of perimenopause and menopause, can be annoying and mentally draining. The Galveston Diet focuses on anti-inflammatory foods that can help control your internal temperature, lowering the frequency and severity of hot flashes. Combating Sleep Disruptions: Sleep problems are another common woe during hormonal changes. The Galveston Diet supports healthy sleep hygiene habits and includes stress-management methods, both of which add to a good night's rest. Additionally, certain anti-inflammatory foods, like tart cherry juice, have been shown to improve sleep quality. Balancing Mood Swings: The chemical changes of perimenopause and menopause can lead to mood swings, anger, and even worry. By improving gut health and lowering inflammation, the Galveston Diet can positively affect mood control. Remember, a healthy gut is often referred to as a "second brain," and the anti-inflammatory foods you eat can affect the production of mood-regulating chemicals.

Supporting Bone Health: Estrogen plays a key part in bone health, and its drop during menopause can increase the risk of osteoporosis. The Galveston Diet includes bone-healthy nutrients like calcium, vitamin D, and magnesium, while also promoting gut health, which is important for optimal calcium intake.

But remember, you're not alone on this trip. Here are some extra tips for handling perimenopause and menopause with the Galveston Diet:

Prioritize Protein: Protein is important for keeping muscle growth and bone health, both of which can be affected by hormonal changes. Include lean protein sources like fish, chicken, beans, and nuts in your diet. Embrace Healthy Fats: Don't shy away from healthy fats like those found in eggs, olive oil, and fatty fish. These fats not only promote satiety but also support hormone production and bone health.

Manage Stress: Chronic stress can cause chemical changes and worsen symptoms. Explore stress-management methods like yoga, meditation, or deep breathing routines.

Seek Support: Don't hesitate to reach out to your healthcare provider or a qualified dietitian for personalized advice throughout perimenopause and menopause.

The Galveston Diet is more than just a collection of meals; it's a mindset of food that allows you to take charge of your health during perimenopause and menopause. By adopting these principles and accepting a complete approach to well-being, you can turn this chemical shift into a song of strength, endurance, and healthy health.

In the next chapter, we'll study how to change the Galveston Diet for individual tastes and food limits. Whether you're vegetarian, gluten-free, or have other dietary needs, we'll provide the tools to build a personal song of food that fits your unique lifestyle. Remember, you are the director of your health, and the Galveston Diet is here to guide you toward a beautiful show throughout life's stages.

Chapter 9: A Symphony of Individuality: Adapting the Galveston Diet for Your Preferences and Needs

The beauty of the Galveston Diet comes in its versatility. It's not a one-size-fits-all method; it's a mindset of food meant to be adapted to your unique tastes and dietary limits. Whether you're a passionate vegetarian seeking plant-based choices, someone with gluten issues managing a restricted diet, or an individual with specific national food traditions, the Galveston Diet can be your peaceful guide to optimal health.

Embracing Vegetarian and Vegan Lifestyles:

For those who have accepted a vegetarian or vegan lifestyle, the Galveston Diet offers a lively symphony of plant-based choices. Here's how to make a healthy and anti-inflammatory veggie or vegan plate:

Protein Powerhouses: Legumes like lentils, chickpeas, and black beans are great sources of plant-based protein. Explore creative ways to add them to your meals, like lentil soups, chickpea stews, or filling bean burgers.

Eggs as Allies: For vegans who include eggs, they can be a useful source of protein and good fats. Enjoy them stirred with spinach and tomatoes, cooked on whole-wheat toast, or combined into veggie omelets packed with bright vegetables.

Dairy options: For those with dairy restrictions, there's a world of wonderful options ready to be discovered. Opt for plain plant-based milks like almond or oat milk for your coffee or shakes. Use coconut milk or cashew cheese as a creamy alternative in recipes.

Navigating Gluten Sensitivities:

If you have gluten allergies, fear not! The Galveston Diet can still be your guide to a symphony of delicious and healthy foods. Here are some tips for a gluten-free adaptation:

Grain Swaps: Instead of wheat-based grains, discover the world of gluten-free choices like quinoa, brown rice, buckwheat, or millet. These nutrient-rich choices provide important carbohydrates without gluten. Label Reading:

Become a label-reading spy! Pay close attention to secret sources of gluten, often found in prepared foods, sauces, and seasonings. Choose goods clearly labeled "gluten-free" to ensure a safe and delicious cooking experience. Get Creative: Don't let gluten restrictions hold you back from loving your favorite meals. Explore gluten-free options for pasta, bread, and baked goods. There's a wealth of delicious meals available online and in cookbooks to satisfy your tastes.

Respecting Cultural Food Traditions:

The Galveston Diet honors and respects the beauty of various ethnic food customs. Here's how to combine your cultural background with the principles of anti-inflammatory nourishment:

Focus on Whole Foods: At the heart of the Galveston Diet lies the focus on whole, raw foods. Explore how classic foods from your culture can be changed using these concepts. Look for ways to add more veggies, lean protein sources, and healthy fats to your meals. Spice Up Your Life: Many countries add a colorful array of spices to their food. Embrace these spices! Many, like turmeric and ginger, hold powerful anti-inflammatory qualities, making them a delicious and health-promoting addition to your meals.

Portion Awareness: Cultural festivals often involve rich and delicious foods. Practice thoughtful eating and amount control to enjoy these special foods while staying in harmony with the principles of the Galveston Diet.

Remember, the Galveston Diet is a path, not a goal. It's about developing a sense of self-awareness and learning to listen to your body's specific needs. By accepting these changes and fostering a spirit of discovery, you can create a personal harmony of nutrition that connects with your tastes and cultural background.

In the next chapter, we'll dive into the exciting world of vitamins and explore their possible role in improving your health within the framework of the Galveston Diet. But before we turn the page, remember: Your identity is your biggest strength. Embrace it, enjoy it, and allow it to guide you on your way to healthy health with the Galveston Diet as your guidance.

Chapter 10: The Energizing Symphony: Exercise for Hormonal Harmony and Vibrant Wellbeing

Imagine a vast concert hall, the orchestra poised, instruments glistening. But the conductor's baton stays motionless. The music, the very soul of the performance, waits to be released. This, my friends, is a metaphor for your body when exercise is omitted from the equation. You possess the magnificent instruments - muscles, lungs, a heart – however without the conductor's call to action, the symphony of health stays mute.

The Galveston Diet has been your guide, painstakingly tuning the instruments of your body via anti-inflammatory nutrients. But for a really great performance, for a life bursting with energy and vitality, we need to add the dynamic conductor – exercise.

Exercise is not simply about shaping muscles or burning calories (although it excels at both!). It's a formidable force for hormonal harmony, a conductor that orchestrates a cascade of favorable changes inside your body. Let's look into the science underlying this profound connection:

The Insulin Tango: Remember the discord produced by insulin resistance in Chapter 7? Exercise functions as a skillful dancing partner, helping your cells become more sensitive to insulin. This smooths the flow of blood sugar, keeping energy levels steady and reducing the undesirable accumulation of extra calories as fat.

The Stress-Busting Beat: Chronic stress may wreak havoc with your hormonal symphony, especially cortisol, the "fight-or-flight" hormone. Exercise functions as a natural stress reliever, stimulating the production of endorphins — your body's feel-good chemicals. This not only improves mood and decreases anxiety, but also helps control cortisol levels, encouraging hormonal equilibrium.

The Estrogen Encore: As we covered in Chapter 8, falling estrogen levels throughout perimenopause and menopause may lead to a cascade of undesirable changes. Exercise, especially weight-bearing activities that encourage bone formation, maybe a strong ally. It helps preserve bone density, decreases the risk of osteoporosis, and may even lessen some of the painful symptoms associated with hormonal shifts. The Sleep Serenade: Struggling with sleep disturbances? Exercise may be your lullaby. Regular physical exercise promotes deeper, more restful sleep, leaving you feeling invigorated and ready to conquer the day.

But how can you include this conductor in your life? Here's a symphony of movement for you to consider:

Find Your Groove: Exercise shouldn't feel like punishment. Explore diverse hobbies - dancing, swimming, hiking, cycling – and find what fuels your delight. When you discover an exercise you like, you're more likely to persist with it in the long term.

Start Slowly and Build: Don't attempt to go from couch potato to marathon runner overnight. Begin with moderate-intensity exercise for 30 minutes most days of the week, gradually increasing the length and intensity as your fitness level increases.

Embrace Strength Training: Don't be afraid of weightlifting! Strength training, even with bodyweight exercises, is vital for growing muscle mass, which not only enhances your physique but also accelerates metabolism and helps control blood sugar levels.

Move Your Body Throughout the Day: Take the stairs instead of the elevator, park farther away from your destination, or perform some stretching exercises throughout your workday. Every ounce of movement matters and adds to the overall symphony of your health.

Remember, you are the master of your health. The Galveston Diet supplied the anti-inflammatory score, and now, with exercise as your conductor, you have the capacity to create a bright and dramatic symphony of well-being. Beauty rests not in reaching perfection, but in the pleasure of movement, the celebration of your body's power and tenacity, and the dedication to a life filled with energy and vitality.

In the following chapter, we'll examine the wonderful realm of sleep and its enormous influence on your health. We'll go into practical techniques to promote a comfortable night's sleep so that your body can really resonate with the harmonic melodies of the Galveston Diet and the exhilarating rhythm of exercise. So, keep flipping the pages, my friends. The melody of your health has just begun!

Chapter 11: The Restorative Symphony: Sleep, Stress Management, and the Galveston Diet Connection

Imagine a world where your body performs at its top, your intellect is clear and focused, and your emotional well-being soars. This, my friends, is the power of a good night's sleep. Sleep isn't a luxury; it's the foundation upon which the symphony of your health is formed. It's the silent maestro that sets the scene for healthy hormone balance, stress reduction, and a powerful immune system. But for many of us, this healing symphony seems like a cacophony of interrupted sleep, restless nights, and the lingering effects of chronic stress.

The good news? The Galveston Diet and excellent stress management practices might be the tools you need to lead a harmonious sleep symphony, leaving you feeling energized and ready to welcome each day. Here's why sleep and stress control are key aspects of the Galveston Diet:

The Hormonal Lullaby: During sleep, your body produces a cascade of hormones, including melatonin, the sleep hormone, and growth hormone, which plays a critical role in cell repair and tissue regeneration. When sleep is interrupted, this hormonal symphony gets out of rhythm, altering everything from metabolism to mood regulation. The Galveston Diet, by supporting anti-inflammatory foods and good eating practices, produces an environment favorable to hormonal balance, opening the path for a more peaceful night's sleep.

The Stress-Busting Serenade: Chronic stress is a renowned sleep robber. The persistent stimulation of the "fight-or-flight" stress response keeps cortisol, the stress hormone, high. This disturbs the regular sleep-wake cycle, making it difficult to fall asleep and remain asleep. By introducing stress-management practices into your routine, like as meditation, deep breathing exercises, or yoga, you may quiet the mind and body, providing a more pleasant atmosphere for sleep.

The Gut-Brain Connection: The gut microbiome, the billions of bacteria resident in your digestive system, has an unexpected function in sleep regulation. The Galveston Diet, with its focus on gut-healthy foods including fermented vegetables and prebiotics, supports a balanced microbiota. This, in turn, may favorably affect the creation of neurotransmitters like serotonin, which adds to feelings of relaxation and well-being, setting the foundation for a good night's sleep.

Now, let's discuss practical techniques to build a pleasant sleep symphony:

Create a Sleep Sanctuary: Transform your bedroom into a refuge for slumber. Ensure it's dark, quiet, and chilly. Invest in blackout curtains, an earplug set, and a comfy mattress that supports your body. Establish a Sleep Schedule: Go to bed and wake up at predictable times, especially on weekends. This helps balance your body's natural sleep-wake cycle. Power Down Before Bed: Avoid displays like TVs, computers, and cell phones for at least an hour before sleep. The blue light generated by these gadgets may interrupt melatonin synthesis and make it difficult to fall asleep. Relaxation Rituals: Develop a peaceful sleep ritual that indicates to your body that it's time to shut down. This may be taking a warm bath, reading a book, or performing gentle stretches.

Mindfulness Practices: Meditation, deep breathing techniques, or progressive muscular relaxation may alleviate anxiety and calm the mind, preparing you for a comfortable sleep.

Remember, stress control is equally vital for sleep harmony. Here are some strategies to consider:

Mindfulness Meditation: Regular meditation practice cultivates a feeling of calm and mindfulness, helping you handle stress in the present and lessen its influence on your sleep.

Deep Breathing Exercises: Simple deep breathing exercises help stimulate the body's relaxation response, decreasing stress hormones and fostering a feeling of tranquility, preparing you for sleep.

Engage in Activities You Enjoy: Make time for activities that offer you pleasure, whether it's spending time in nature, listening to music, or pursuing a hobby. These hobbies may help relieve stress and enhance emotions of well-being.

Seek Support: Don't be hesitant to seek professional treatment if you're battling with chronic stress or sleep difficulties. A therapist may give helpful information and strategies to manage stress and enhance your sleep quality.

By adopting the concepts of the Galveston Diet, implementing efficient stress-management practices, and emphasizing good sleep habits, you may lead a symphony of restful sleep. It's a symphony that will resound well beyond the bedroom, altering your energy levels, emotions, cognitive function, and general well-being.

As you flip the page to the next chapter, remember this: A good night's sleep is not a luxury; it's necessary for maximum health. With the Galveston Diet as your guide and a dedication to stress management, you may create the optimal atmosphere for a peaceful and rejuvenating sleep.

Chapter 12: Living a Vibrant Life: Beyond Diet and Exercise—The Symphony of Wholeness

The Galveston Diet has been your guide, leading you through the delicate motions of anti-inflammatory nutrition. Exercise has emerged as your dynamic maestro, conducting a symphony of hormonal balance and physical well-being. But a really robust existence goes beyond nutrition and exercise. It's about fostering a feeling of completeness by engaging in behaviors that benefit your mind, body, and soul. It's all about finding your own unique instruments and learning to play them in beautiful harmony.

Power of Positive Relationships: Human connection is more than a social nicety; it is an essential component of a fulfilling existence. Strong, supportive connections provide a feeling of belonging, love, and purpose. They reduce the effects of stress, enhance happiness, and may even strengthen your immune system. Invest in sustaining your relationships with loved ones, whether it means spending quality time with family, reconnecting with old acquaintances, or making new connections in your community.

Find Your Flow: Flow is the euphoric condition of total immersion in an activity, in which time seems to melt away and you feel pure pleasure and contentment. It may be found in a wide range of hobbies, including painting, singing, dancing, gardening, and carpentry. When you find activities that enable you to reach this state of flow, you not only foster creativity and self-expression, but you also enjoy an increase in endorphins, the body's natural feel-good hormones.

Embracing gratitude: Gratitude is more than simply a transient emotion; it is a powerful discipline that may shift your perspective and improve your overall well-being. Take time each day, whether via blogging or silent thought, to enjoy the positive things in your life, such as the sun's warmth on your skin, laughter shared with a loved one, or the basic act of breathing. By practicing thankfulness, you redirect your emphasis to the good elements of life, promoting satisfaction and optimism.

Give Back to the World: There's an evident delight in assisting others. Volunteering your time and skills for a cause you care about helps your community while also providing a feeling of purpose and connection. Giving back, whether by mentoring a kid, volunteering at an animal shelter, or participating in a neighborhood clean-up initiative, enables you to contribute to something larger than yourself, promoting a feeling of contentment and well-being.

Living With Purpose: A flourishing existence is based on purpose. What drives your passion? What kind of legacy are you hoping to leave? Finding your mission does not have to be a tremendous job. It might be as easy as wanting to be the greatest version of yourself every day or rekindling a long-dormant creative passion. When you live with purpose, you wake up every morning with a feeling of direction and determination, adding a lovely tune to your life's symphony.

Remember: this is a journey, not a destination. There may be times when your symphony seems dissonant, when obstacles occur and tension threatens to drown out the melody. But that is the beauty of a symphony: it is distinguished not by its faultless notes, but by its capacity to overcome discord and produce harmony using a variety of instruments. Embrace the road, celebrate your accomplishments, and don't be afraid to explore and find out what actually makes your life vibrate with pleasure and meaning.

The Galveston Diet has enabled you to take control of your health and become the master of your own well-being. It has given you the resources you need to fuel your body with anti-inflammatory foods, exercise your body joyfully, and prioritize restorative sleep. But beyond these components is a huge universe waiting to be discovered. Accept the habits that benefit your mind, body, and soul. Cultivate good connections, find your rhythm, and live with purpose. This beautiful convergence - the symphony of sustenance, activity, relaxation, connection, and purpose - reveals the full potential for a robust and meaningful existence. So, my reader, keep turning the pages of your life's narrative. Let the music play! The world eagerly awaits your one-of-a-kind and exquisite symphony.

Conclusion: The Galveston Diet—A Grand Crescendo on Your Journey to Wholeness

We've reached the end of this transformational adventure. As you finish this book, you will see the Galveston Diet as more than simply a collection of recipes or a rigorous set of rules, but as a strong compass directing you to a healthier, happier life. It has been your companion in navigating the complex realm of inflammation and its influence on your health. It has given you the ability to be the conductor of your hormonal symphony, bringing harmony via the power of anti-inflammatory nutrition.

However, the Galveston Diet is more than simply a food strategy. It's a way of life, an invitation to embrace a comprehensive symphony of well-being. Throughout these pages, we've looked at the profound link between activity and hormonal balance, the restorative effect of sleep, and the value of cultivating a stress-free mind. We've discussed the value of great connections, the delight of finding your flow, and the importance of living with purpose.

This adventure, however, has not ended. It's just the beginning. As you leave these pages, bring the spirit of the Galveston Diet with you. Remember that the greatest profound changes often occur beyond the pages of a book. Accept the kitchen as a creative environment, where you may experiment with anti-inflammatory products and create culinary masterpieces that feed both your body and spirit. Allow your body to move with delight, whether it's a brisk stroll in nature, a dance party in your living room, or the exciting challenge of a new physical activity. Prioritize restorative sleep, establish a relaxing environment, and build good sleeping habits.

The route to a flourishing life is not linear. There will be times when your symphony seems dissonant, when cravings develop, or when stress knocks you off balance. Remember, the beauty of a symphony is its capacity to overcome discord and generate harmony from a variety of instruments. Accept these problems as chances for progress, such as learning to listen to your body's specific demands and fine-tuning your internal symphony.

The Galveston Diet has provided you with the information and skills you need to manage these situations. You've learned how to understand the language of inflammation, identify your emotional triggers, and make intelligent eating choices. You've found the transformational power of exercise, the restorative enchantment of sleep, and the value of taking a holistic approach to well-being.

As you continue, keep in mind that you are the conductor of your own health symphony. You have the ability to build a life full of robust energy, hormonal balance, and profound happiness. Let the Galveston Diet serve as your guide and compass on this fantastic trip to a better, happier self. Most importantly, enjoy the trip. Enjoy the pleasures of tasty and healthy meals, appreciate your body's strength and resilience through activity, and value the restorative benefits of a good night's sleep.

Remember that living a lively life is not about attaining perfection; it is about embracing your inner music, playing each note with purpose, and building a symphony that reflects your unique beat. So, my reader, keep turning the pages of your life's narrative. Allow the melody of the Galveston Diet to play on, creating a symphony of well-being that inspires not just yourself but everyone around you. The world eagerly awaits your lovely and lively music.

Appendix: Sample Meal Plans and Recipes—A Culinary Adventure with the Galveston Diet

Welcome to the delicious world of the Galveston Diet! This appendix acts as your culinary compass, providing a range of example meal plans and delectable dishes to help you get started on your anti-inflammatory journey. Remember, these are just the beginning points. Feel free to experiment, switch items according to your tastes, and let your inner chef shine!

Sample Meal Plan 1: A Day of Vivacious Breakfast, Lunch, and Dinner

Breakfast (Nourishing and Energizing): Creamy Chia Seed Pudding with Berries and Sliced Almonds: This fiber-rich pudding gives prolonged energy, while the berries provide antioxidants. To add some healthy fats, top it with sliced almonds.

Recipe: Mix 1/4 cup chia seeds with 1 cup unsweetened almond or coconut milk. Add 1 teaspoon of honey (optional) and a sprinkle of vanilla extract. Refrigerate overnight. In the morning, garnish with fresh berries and sliced almonds.

For a light and flavorful lunch, try the Mediterranean Chickpea Salad Sandwich on Whole-Wheat Bread. This protein-packed salad is full of flavor and keeps you satiated.

Recipe: Toss cooked chickpeas with chopped red onion, diced cucumber, crumbled feta cheese, chopped fresh parsley, and a lemon vinaigrette dressing. Serve with whole wheat bread.

Dinner options include salmon with roasted vegetables and lemon quinoa. Season salmon fillets with olive oil, salt, and pepper for a balanced meal that includes protein, healthy fats, and complex carbs. Roast in the oven with chopped veggies such as broccoli, carrots, and bell peppers. Cook the quinoa according to package directions and fluff with a splash of lemon juice.

Sample Meal Plan 2: A Vegetarian Delight

For a sweet and satisfying breakfast, try whole-wheat pancakes with berries and maple syrup drizzle. Enjoy a healthier spin on a traditional breakfast.

To make a batter, combine whole wheat flour, baking powder, salt, and unsweetened plant-based milk. Fry the pancakes on a griddle that has been gently oiled. Add fresh berries and a sprinkle of maple syrup.

Lunch (Light and Refreshing): - Lentil Salad with Chopped Vegetables and a Lemon Herb Dressing: Packed with protein, fiber, and refreshing tastes. Recipe: Cook lentils according to package directions. Combine with diced cucumbers, cherry tomatoes, and red onions. Make a dressing with olive oil, lemon juice, chopped fresh herbs (such as parsley or mint), and a touch of salt and pepper. Toss everything together and enjoy.

Warm and flavorful vegetarian chili with kidney beans, black beans, and corn is ideal for a nice night in. To prepare, sauté chopped onions, bell peppers, and garlic in olive oil. Combine chopped tomatoes, kidney beans, black beans, corn, vegetable broth, chili powder, cumin, and a sprinkle of smoky paprika. Simmer for thirty minutes. Add a dollop of plain Greek yogurt and sliced avocado for added richness.

Recipe Showcase: A Look at Delicious Possibilities

This section provides an overview of the gastronomic pleasures that await you on your Galveston Diet excursion.

Spiced Turmeric Chicken with Roasted Brussels Sprouts This recipe is a brilliant burst of flavor, with turmeric providing anti-inflammatory benefits. To make a hearty supper, roast Brussels sprouts till soft and combine with turmeric-seasoned chicken breast. Coconut Curry Lentil Soup. This soothing soup is high in protein and fiber. Sauté veggies such as onions, carrots, and bell peppers in coconut oil. Combine the lentils, vegetable broth, curry powder, and coconut milk. Simmer until lentils are soft. Season with lime juice and fresh cilantro. Baked Salmon with Herbs and Lemon Butter Sauce: This exquisite recipe is ideal for a special occasion. Bake salmon fillets seasoned with fresh herbs such as rosemary and thyme. Top with a light and tasty lemon butter sauce prepared from melted butter, lemon juice, and chopped fresh parsley.

These are just a few ideas to spark your culinary imagination. Remember that the Galveston Diet promotes discovery! Experiment with various products, spices, and cooking methods to create nutritious and tasty meals that appeal to your specific taste.

Embrace the journey Beyond the Recipes

This appendix is more than simply a compilation of recipes; it's an invitation to rediscover the pleasure of cooking. Here are some extra suggestions to make your culinary trip with the Galveston Diet even more enjoyable:

 Plan Your Meals: Planning your meals ahead of time ensures that you always have nutritious alternatives accessible.

If this book was enjoyable, please write a review.

Thank you for embarking
on this transforming
journey with us!" here is
your free gift!

Scan the above QR
code to get your free
gift!